2 cD

The British School of Osteopathy

and Listening

ations

A MODERN APPROACH

Talking and Listening to Patients

A MODERN APPROACH

Professor C. M. FLETCHER

CBE, MD, FRCP

Emeritus Professor of Clinical
Epidemiology, University of London

AND

Professor PAUL FREELING

OBE, FRCGP

Professor of General Practice and
Head of the Department of General Practice
and Primary Care, St George's Hospital
Medical School

The Nuffield Provincial Hospitals Trust

Published by the
Nuffield Provincial Hospitals Trust
3 Prince Albert Road, London NW1 7SP

ISBN 0 900574 70 4

© Nuffield Provincial Hospitals Trust 1988

Designed by Bernard Crossland
Typeset in Modern Light
and printed in Great Britain by
Burgess & Son (Abingdon) Ltd
Abingdon, Oxfordshire

Contents

APPENDICES

Foreword

In 1972 the Nuffield Provincial Hospitals Trust published in its Rock Carling Monograph Series *Communication in Medicine* by C. M. Fletcher. In the subsequent six years the Trust became increasingly concerned with the practical consequences of failures of communication in the National Health Service, and in particular with improving communication between doctors and patients. It was clear that this was often seriously deficient so that many patients were dissatisfied with the information they were given and ignored the advice they received. A series of seminars held during that period reviewed research on this subject, little of which had been reported in journals commonly read by doctors. Since much of that work had been concerned with methods by which medical students could be more effectively taught skills of communication, the Trust set up a working party to produce a short account for medical teachers of recent developments in this field and this was published in 1978, *Talking with Patients: a teaching approach*. Fifty copies were sent to each medical school. Subsequent sales of three reprints of the booklet and the fact that several medical schools still provide a copy for each of their clinical students show that it proved useful.

In the 10 years since the first edition appeared, there have been important advances in this subject. Although it has become more widely recognized as necessary for the successful practice of clinical medicine it is still allocated little time in the curricula of most medical schools. Therefore it was decided to prepare a revised and fuller edition. Professor Charles Fletcher and Professor Paul Freeling were invited to undertake this. The text was circulated to most of the members of the original working party and also to Dr D. Tuckett and Dr D. Pendleton, and their suggestions were incorporated. The final text was agreed by the chairman, Sir John Walton.

In the first edition, common faults of doctors were satirized in cartoons. It is now felt that a more positive approach is needed, picking out some of the cardinal points in what is virtually a short textbook on how more effective exchange of information between doctors and those who seek their help in clinical consultations may be achieved.

Introduction

Despite all the recent technical developments in medicine, the consultation remains the indispensable unit of medical practice (1). Its success depends on how well doctors and patients communicate with each other, so that the doctor obtains a full insight into the patient's problems and the patient is enabled to understand and accept the doctor's conclusions and advice. The first part of the consultation can aptly be described as the **'interview'**; but the word 'exposition' used in the first edition to describe the second part seems rather inappropriate, for it suggests that doctors need do no more than tell patients about their conclusions. It is now well recognized that doctors need to take account of the patient's own views about their illness and expectations. They can then negotiate an agreed conclusion on diagnosis and management which patients can accept as appropriate solutions to the problems which have led them to consult a doctor. We now propose the word **'discussion'** for this part of the consultation. This altered view of the consultation is consistent with the current trend in medical ethics away from the traditional paternalism of doctors and towards encouraging patients' autonomy.

Another advance since the first edition of this booklet has been the emphasis given to communication skills in vocational training for primary care. More attention is now being given in several medical schools to teaching better interviewing of patients, but there is seldom any teaching about the discussion. There appears to be no teaching of communication skills in the postgraduate training of specialists other than psychiatrists (2).

One reason for this contrast may be found in two major studies of communication skills in general practice. In 1976 Byrne and Long (3) showed that a frequent reason for patients' dissatisfaction with their consultations was that many doctors had such limited interviewing skills that they sometimes failed even to find out the main reason why patients had come to see them. In 1985 Tuckett *et al* (4) reported extensive studies of such consultations, and, with special attention to the discussions, showed how more satisfactory outcomes might be achieved. No similar studies of consultants' communication skills in hospital clinics have been published, but in one study of young hospital doctors (5) serious defects, especially in giving information, were found and it was suggested that these deficiencies were likely to persist throughout their careers in the absence of any further tuition, which they are unlikely ever to receive (2).

Hospital doctors' communication needs may be thought to differ from those of the general practitioner in that most hospital patients are referred for investigation of and advice on predetermined clinical problems, while the GP has to look beyond the patient's presenting symptoms to discover their origins—which may be physical, social, or emotional in various proportions. Nonetheless both the consultant and GP may give unacceptable advice if the patient's view of his illness and its psycho-social aspects are not elucidated and taken into account, for these may be as important to many patients as their physical illnesses. Thus there are few essential differences between the communication skills needed in these two areas of clinical practice.

This booklet will briefly review, in the light of these and other studies, the reasons for failures of communication in both parts of a consultation. It will describe teaching methods which may help both students and their teachers to recognize how their communication with patients could be bettered, and will make suggestions for research which is still much needed in this field.

The *Interview*

At first most students have some difficulty in talking to patients about their illnesses. They used to get little instruction about how to interview them other than being given lists of questions to ask in order to clarify patients' initial complaints and to ensure that no other important symptoms had been missed. Such questions are needed, but only in moderation. A barrage of routine questions can seriously inhibit communication.

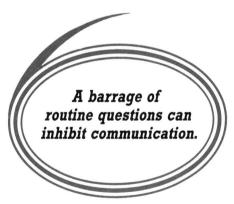

A barrage of routine questions can inhibit communication.

In the course of the clinical years, students' interviewing skills may actually deteriorate rather than improve (6,7). Before they have acquired much medical knowledge, they listen to what patients have to tell them, expressing concern about their emotional reactions to their illnesses and their social difficulties. When they have learnt more about diseases their attitude changes owing to their perception of their teachers' main interests. They then tend to make a quick, provisional diagnosis of physical illness, and to confine the patient to answering questions which appear relevant to it. If this happens to be wrong or incomplete their conclusions will also be faulty. Moreover, students know that in their final clinical examination they will usually be expected only to reach a simple diagnosis of physical disease. Some examiners actually reprove candidates for wasting time on 'irrelevant' psycho-social issues.

When they have qualified, most retain this bias against discovering patients' anxieties about illnesses and their emotional and social consequences (4,5,8–13), even though these may be as important in caring for them as are the physical manifestations for which a simple 'history taking' approach can provide an accurate diagnosis (14).

After a few years of clinical practice most doctors think they are good at interviewing, but this assumption was certainly not true of most of the GPs' interviews studied by Byrne and Long (3). They tended to use an inquisitorial or 'doctor centred' style in which the doctor did most of the talking: only a minority of the interviews were 'patient centred' with the doctors talking less and listening to what their patients wished to tell them, not only about their symptoms but also about their psycho-social problems. The young hospital doctors studied in Manchester were also disinclined to find out about such problems (5).

Importance of good interviewing skills

A correct and full diagnosis of both physical illness and any associated or causative emotional and social problems is essential for good management. In primary health care many patients come to consultations with their own ideas of what is wrong with them and what should be done about it. Any ideas which are false must be discovered and corrected if the patient is to accept and act on the doctor's advice. Patients are often anxious that they may

A complete diagnosis, physical and psycho-social depends on the skill of the interviewer.

have a serious disease; if this anxiety is not detected and eased, it will persist. Moreover some patients who really need help with a personal problem hesitate to mention it, but present some minor symptom as an excuse for seeking their doctor's help. An interview which concentrates on this symptom and ignores the real problem will result in irrelevant, or at least inadequate, management. Students must learn to conduct efficient interviews if they are to become skilled clinicians.

Learning good interviewing

STRATEGY

The doctor has three purposes. First, to diagnose any physical illness; second, to elucidate any anxieties which patients may have about their symptoms and circumstances and third, to discover whether they have any ideas of their own about diagnosis, prognosis, or treatment. The usual process is for the doctor to form a hypothesis to account for the history, presenting symptoms, and emotional aspects of the patient's illness and by further questioning to confirm, refute, or modify it. It is tested further by physical examination and, in some cases, special investigations or referral to a specialist. When a hypothesis is found to be wrong others are formed and tested in the same way (15).

A MODEL

The first essential is to have a clear idea of the best form of an interview. A precis of an admirable model, devised by Maguire and Rutter (16), is given in Appendix 1. It may be found useful to duplicate this for students, with any modification which individual teachers may wish to make. This may help them, but they will still have to acquire the skills needed to apply the model successfully.

SKILLS

These are really no more than modifications of the social skills that are used by anyone who has to find out about other people efficiently, such as reporters, employers, and other professionals. Some people are naturally good at this; others may find it difficult, at least in special circumstances or with particular types of people. The skills needed for good interviewing are listed in Table 1. The most important of these is to listen perceptively to what the patient is trying to say.

At present many students are just given a list of questions to ask but are taught little else about interviewing. They cannot copy their teachers, for they seldom see them interviewing patients. There are now several good video-tapes which demonstrate skills required in the interview and difficulties which may be met*. But, however well a student may come to understand how a clinical interview should be conducted, he is sure to encounter some difficulties and it is hard for him to know how well he is doing. The most effective teaching method is for students to watch video recordings of their own interviews

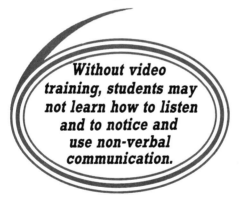

Without video training, students may not learn how to listen and to notice and use non-verbal communication.

so that they can see themselves as their patients see them. Without video teaching it is difficult for students to learn the importance of noticing and using non-verbal communication. Discussion of these tapes with a tutor (and/or with fellow students) helps them to see how to

---

* MSD Foundation, Tavistock House, Tavistock Square, London WC1H 9LG.

TABLE 1

Skills needed for good interviewing

1. Beginning the interview

- (a) Arrange seating so that doctor and patient are conveniently close—not separated by a desk.
- (b) Give friendly greeting with self-introduction.
- (c) Show empathy and warmth.

2. Explain interview's:

- (a) Purpose, to discover patient's problems.
- (b) Need for precision.
- (c) Need for note taking.
- (d) Time available.

Check that patient is happy about all this.

3. Obtaining information

- (a) Use open questions:
  'Do you have . . .? rather than 'You don't have . . .do you?'
- (b) Facilitate
  verbal: 'Go on', 'Tell me more'.
  non-verbal: nodding and looking attentive.
- (c) Listen
  don't interrupt, except for irrelevances. don't ask next question before full answer to last one has been given.
- (d) Accept silence
  while patient is hesitating or thinking what to say.
- (e) Recognize
  irrelevance and get back to the point.
- (f) Clarify
  details of symptoms and of any medical terms used by doctor or patient.
- (g) Observe patient
  for important clues, verbal or non-verbal.
- (h) Tolerate
  emotionally distasteful aspects of the story without appearing shocked.
- (i) Summarize
  patient's problems both in the course of the interview and at the end: checking that you have got them right.

become more skilful. Not only have students themselves found this method helpful, but it has been clearly shown in several studies (17–19) that video-tape teaching results in a highly significant improvement in students' skills compared with those acquired by control students taught by conventional methods. It has now been shown that these improved skills persist after students qualify and start to practice (5). Surgical patients have been found to rate students who have acquired these skills as more empathic and understanding than those who lack them (20).

Without video teaching it is difficult for students to learn the importance of noticing, and using, non-verbal communication. They may be helped by using standard marking sheets (17,18) to rate their own and their fellow students' competence, while watching video-tapes of their interviews. These recorded interviews can be done with co-operative patients or with actors, who can simulate patients extremely well (5), and can comment usefully on how well the student seems to them to be performing.

Teachers may feel that, if they are to teach effective interviewing, they must first be confident of their own skills. It could be helpful if teachers were to take an ordinary audio-recorder into one of their out-patient clinics to record

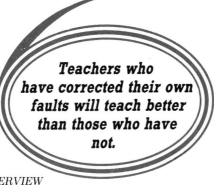

Teachers who have corrected their own faults will teach better than those who have not.

their own interviews, and subsequently to listen to them so that they can see what faults they had been making and how they could be corrected (21). Teachers who have discovered and corrected their own faults are likely to teach better than those who have not.

If an interview is to be well conducted doctors must have, and must show by their manner, a real interest in and understanding of patients as people and not just as interesting examples of patho-physiology. There is no better way of discouraging patients from giving a full account of their illnesses than by looking bored or by concentrating on note-taking. Some patients say, after a consultation: 'The doctor never even looked at me'. Such apparent lack of interest may be given quite unintentionally by students, but are obvious to them when they see a video-tape of themselves with a patient, and are usually easily corrected. Some teachers who have used video-tape recordings, however, find that a small proportion of students do not improve their interviewing skills. They seem to find it difficult to develop any real affinity with patients or to put them at their ease. It is important to identify such students; for they may need counselling or special training. If this is ineffective they should perhaps be advised to enter some non-clinical branch of medicine.

ENQUIRING ABOUT EMBARRASSING PROBLEMS

Doctors' interviewing differs from that of other professions in that it often, if not usually, involves topics which are embarrassing to the patient and sometimes to themselves. When such matters come up in a consultation the doctor must not show any discomfiture which could inhibit the patient from being frank. Nowadays excretory functions can usually be discussed quite openly, but sexual activities,

Learning good interviewing

despite modern liberalism, may be felt too intimate by doctor or patient for easy discussion, particularly when they concern sexual practices which the doctor finds disturbing. All doctors must learn how to handle such matters calmly. Formerly, sexual problems were never referred to in medical education, and even now they may not be brought up for candid discussion with students in their clinical course. If doctors are to help their patients with their emotional problems, which often have a sexual basis, they must learn from their teachers how to encourage their patients to talk about them and to know what they can handle themselves and what they should refer on to experts. Seminars on sexuality, arranged so that students can drop their defences and discuss their inhibitions, should be provided in all medical schools (22,23).

TIME

One necessity for effective interviewing is efficient use of time. Waste of time may be avoided by quick discovery of patients' main problems and by keeping them to the point. In many simple cases of common disorders only a few minutes may be needed to elicit the relevant facts, discover the patients' views and explain the treatment with the help of a pamphlet (see p. 59). Patients will not feel rushed by doctors who show interest in them and concern about what they say. The time which most GP's allocate to each patient in their appointment systems is 7–10 minutes. Tuckett, *et al* (4) found no relationship between the amount of time doctors spent on finding out about patients' views and the length of their consultations: moreover, knowledge of patients' views could reduce time wasted on enquiring about symptoms that are unrelated to patients' real problems. With some patients, especially where

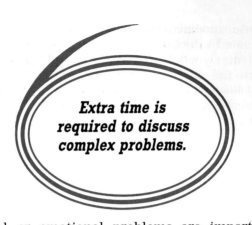

Extra time is required to discuss complex problems.

social or emotional problems are important, more time is needed to acquire a deep enough understanding to be able to counsel a patient properly. But for the main purpose of the interview, which is to make a diagnosis, fifteen minutes is usually long enough with medical patients in hospital practice. For surgical patients less time may be necessary. Good interviews may on average take longer than less good ones (15,24) but if this means that they are more effective they will save time in the long run. Additional time required for some patients may be arranged for a subsequent consultation. Some hospital doctors have found it helpful to send their patients a questionnaire about symptoms when their out-patient appointments are confirmed. They find this saves time otherwise spent on asking routine questions. A blank space can also be provided in which the patient can note 'any other matters you would like to discuss with the doctor' (25). This can reveal problems which might have been overlooked. Such problems may sometimes be confided to a clinic nurse or a receptionist, who should always be encouraged by doctors to tell them anything they have discovered which the doctor should know.

Psycho-social problems, which are too often neglected (8–13), are important in many patients. Good interviewing should not only discover them, but elicit all the relevant data. Its aim is to reach as complete a diagnosis as possible on which to base effective management.

The *Discussion*

The word discussion rather than exposition is used to describe the second part of a consultation. This is because doctors should not just tell patients about the diagnosis and proposals for management, but should first find out their views and discuss them in order to reach an agreed diagnosis and plan of action. Patients will be more likely to accept and carry out this plan if they have participated in its formulation (4,15,26). Bodley Scott (27) described the discussion as 'the doctor's quintessential function, for it is a necessary preliminary to any treatment, nevertheless,' he continued 'we seldom discuss it with our students and never instruct them in its management'. This neglect in teaching has persisted. In 1981 a study of young doctors' communication skills (5) found that few of them were competent in the discussion. They blamed

A study of young doctors' consultations found that few were competent at the discussion.

their incompetence, of which they were aware, on never having been taught how to do it.

Evidence of discussion failures

There is ample evidence of patients' frequent dissatisfaction with what doctors tell them about their illnesses both in general and in hospital practice (28–31). More serious is the fact that many patients do not do what their doctors think they have told them to do. In various studies it has been found that between 10 and 70 per cent of patients (average 50 per cent) do not take their prescribed medicines and reject their doctor's advice about changes in life-style (31,32). Taking a conservative estimate that in Britain 30 per cent of prescribed drugs are not taken or are incorrectly taken, it may be estimated that some £900m is wasted in the NHS every year as a result of poor communication. Much of this loss could be avoided, and treatment made more effective, if doctors learnt to communicate better with patients about their treatment as some GPs have shown is possible (33).

Reasons for discussion failures

1. DOCTORS' ATTITUDES

Many doctors used to think it was bad for patients to understand their illnesses and treatment. 'Good patients' did what they were told without question: 'troublesome' ones questioned doctors in a way which was thought to undermine respect for, and confidence in, their doctors (34). Even now there are some who still adopt this old-fashioned notion. Despite the

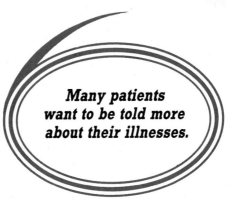

Many patients want to be told more about their illnesses.

change from this attitude towards liberal information, many patients do still find it difficult to get all the information they want about their illnesses, and they are not invited, as they would wish, to take part in deciding about their treatment. Some patients, of course, do not want to participate in decision-making: they need absolute, uncritical confidence in their doctors' skills and prefer not to be pestered with too much information. But several studies have shown that most patients do want more information than they are given (28–31). They wish to know at least why they have become ill and what their diagnosis implies. They also want to take some part in deciding about their treatment in the light of its chances of success and any unpleasant side effects which it may cause. A skilful doctor will achieve the correct balance between autonomy and paternalism for each patient.

2. DOCTORS' DIFFICULTIES WITH GIVING INFORMATION

The main reason for this, as mentioned above, is their having had no formal teaching as students about how to give information and advice to patients in ways which they will understand and accept. This may also be due in part to some teachers under-rating patients' needs for information about their illnesses. Although the model for good interviewing and the necessary skills which are given in Table 1 is now widely accepted, there was no model for the discussion until quite recently. Pendleton's group (15) defined seven tasks for a consultation of which tasks 3–5 deal with giving information, deciding on actions to deal with the present problems, and prevention of recurrences. Appendix 2 provides a model for a discussion. It is more elaborate than that of the Pendleton group because discussions can have many forms. It is intended to be comprehensive while they dealt with discussions only in general practice.

3. PATIENTS' FAILURE TO TAKE IN WHAT THE DOCTOR IS SAYING

This is seldom due to inattention for, except when bad news has to be given, patients want to follow what doctors tell them, but they are often

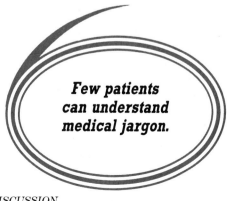

Few patients can understand medical jargon.

confused by doctors using the sort of jargon which they habitually use with their colleagues, forgetting that few patients can understand it (35–37). It may also be because their own ideas about their anatomy and bodily functions are so different from reality that they cannot follow what the doctor is saying. If patients' attention seems to be wandering, it may be because they are confused, and doctors should ask them to repeat back to them what has just been said. Patients sometimes give extraordinary accounts of what they think doctors have told them. Asher (39) described a lady who assured him that 'the house physician had provided her with a new medicine consisting of a strong solution of rubber dissolved in orangeade which was designed to fill up the cracks in the ulcer and set'. This purpose she said 'had been achieved'. If that house physician had asked the patient to repeat to him what she thought he had said she might have got a clearer idea about her treatment.

Nowadays a serious consequence of misunderstanding occurs when a patient has seen a technical report on an investigation which shows a marginal abnormality, and assumes that it will have dire consequences (40). This problem may become commoner when patients have easy access to their clinical records.

4. SHORTAGE OF TIME

Inevitably doctors are often rushed. Good communication demands that they should not appear to their patients to be in a hurry. Few things are more daunting to patients than to have a doctor who appears to be, or worse still, is too busy to be concerned about their problems. When they are short of the time which is necessary for any discussion, it is best not to give a cursory opinion, but to specify a later time when they can give full attention to the patient's problems and answer any question he or she wants to ask. The next section will discuss ways to improve understanding whilst saving time.

5. INAPPROPRIATE ADVICE
OR PRESCRIPTIONS

Doctors who have not conducted good interviews may well misunderstand their patients' needs. Before starting an interview about the symptom first mentioned by the patient it is worth asking: 'Is there anything else you want us to talk about?' Advice about the wrong problem is obviously a waste of time. So is an inappropriate prescription. A patient with a headache which is due to worry about a difficult child will not take a prescribed analgesic, for she knows it will not help. Nor will patients use a medicine against which they have prejudices which the doctor has failed to discover.

Prescribing several medicines with instructions to take them at various intervals before or after food makes it almost impossible for even the most co-operative patient to use them correctly.

What can be done to improve the discussion?

---

1. BETTER TEACHING OF
THE DISCUSSION

Teaching of the discussion, hitherto neglected, must take account of recent ideas which have been developed chiefly from studies of consultations in primary care (4,15). No study of discussion skills of hospital consultants, who do most of the teaching of students, has yet been published. It could be most helpful if some of these teachers were to take part in similar studies of their own skills. They might then see more clearly how to teach their students to conduct better discussions.

Meanwhile, in all clinical teaching the social and psychological impact of illnesses on patients, at present often neglected in hospital (8–13) should be considered, as well as what patients do know and should know about their illnesses and their treatment. When audit sessions are held on discharged patients the information they received before discharge and whether they understood it should be discussed (41).

2. TAKING ACCOUNT OF PATIENTS' VIEWS ON THEIR PROBLEMS

Although included by Maguire and Rutter (16) in their model of the interview, this has not yet been widely recognized as necessary for a good discussion. Many patients come to their doctors

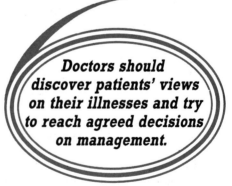

Doctors should discover patients' views on their illnesses and try to reach agreed decisions on management.

with more or less precise ideas, often quite wrong, about what is wrong with them, its causes and what should be done about it. Some patients have idiosyncratic health beliefs which may need to be considered in relation to their willingness to comply with treatment (42). Some are afraid that they have serious disease. To be effective, doctors should discover patients' own ideas about their problems and aim to modify them, if necessary, in the light of biomedical knowledge so as to reach agreed rational decisions on how best to handle their problems (4,15,26). If these are the outcomes of discussions, patients are more likely than they would otherwise have been, to be relieved of any inappropriate anxiety and to adopt effective management. This is the purpose of the consultation which can also, when appropriate, be combined with health education (p. 48).

This concept of a discussion is not one which is readily accepted by doctors who have been trained to appear authoritarian to ignorant patients and to ordain what they should do by 'doctors' orders'. Such attitudes may have been all right when society sanctioned them, when patients were much less well educated and when doctors had, in any case, few effective remedies to offer so that non-compliance did not matter. Since patients want doctors to like them, they are slow to risk giving offence by disagreeing with them. So doctors must take the initiative in encouraging them to voice contrary views. As this comes to be done more often in consultations, patients will respond by being more ready to share their ideas with doctors. Today friendly co-operation between doctor and patient based on mutual respect should promote therapeutic success.

A few patients may come to see their doctors without any idea of what may be wrong with them, just wanting to be told what they should do: but doctors should check that this is so and then make sure that they have understood and will carry out the advice that they have been given.

3. ENCOURAGING PATIENTS' QUESTIONS

A corollary to the need to discover patients' views is to encourage them to ask questions to which they want answers, but hesitate to ask. Many patients come away from a consultation with doubts and questions which they had not mentioned because they thought they should not bother the doctor with them (4,43). Doctors should deliberately make it easy for their patients to ask such questions; for answering them may remove anxieties or misconceptions of which the doctor is unaware, and to answer them will increase the educational function of the consultation. It may help if doctors provide simple pamphlets or notices in their waiting rooms making it clear that they would like to answer any questions that patients want to ask them.

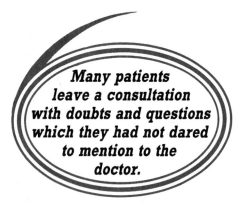

Many patients leave a consultation with doubts and questions which they had not dared to mention to the doctor.

After a consultation some patients think of questions they meant but forgot to ask. A system allowing for some brief appointments should make it easier for such patients to come and get the answers they want.

4. BETTER VERBAL INFORMATION

The main topics about which a doctor may have to inform each patient include: diagnosis (the causes of the patient's problems), treatment, prognosis, how to prevent any recurrence and what social or psychological consequences of the illness there may be and how to cope with them. Very few of the GPs studied by Tuckett *et al* (4) nor any of the young doctors studied in Manchester (5) mentioned all of these topics and few were judged to have spoken clearly about those that they did mention. This is not surprising since none of these doctors had had any training on how to discuss their findings with patients. But this does show how important it is that such training should be undertaken in all medical schools.

Ley (31) concluded, from many studies of patients' recollections of what they had been told by doctors, that this could be improved if the doctors used simple language, and repeated their advice, giving specific rather than general advice, e.g. 'You must lose 12 lbs of weight', rather than 'You must lose weight'.

5. PRINTED OR RECORDED INFORMATION

It is strange, in view of the time factor, that so few doctors use printed or recorded information to supplement what they tell their patients. The amount of information that patients may need is much more than there is time to give verbally during most consultations. This is particularly true of prescriptions (Appendix 2). As a consequence most patients are found to know little about the purposes of their medicines, how to take and store them, or what to do if they seem not to be doing any good, or are producing unpleasant side effects. All of this they need and want to know (44).

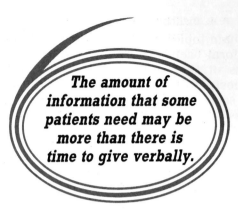

The amount of information that some patients need may be more than there is time to give verbally.

Studies in the USA (45) and recently in this country (46,47) have shown that patient satisfaction, understanding and compliance can be significantly increased by skilfully designed leaflets issued with their prescriptions. In the near future the manufacturers intend to provide such leaflets incorporated in all medicine packages, but doctors will still need to encourage patients to read them and to ensure that someone will convey their content to the illiterate, the blind, and those who do not understand English.

Simple explanations of many diseases are issued by patients' associations and these should be made available, at least for commoner diseases, in surgeries, clinics, and hospital wards. Lists of such associations are available for these and for many less common conditions (48,49). Patients with chronic diseases in whose management they have to play a major role should be encouraged to join the relevant association.

Surgical patients can often be helped to understand what will be done to them by simple diagrams (36). One orthopaedic surgeon made audio-tape recordings of simple accounts of the nature and post-operative care of operations he performed. After an out-patient clinic or an admission to his ward his patients were provided with a recorder in order to listen to the relevant tape. This encouraged them to ask questions about anything they had not understood (50). These recordings were much appreciated and wider use should be made of this method. Such recordings could also be valuable in ensuring truly informed consent to operations. When asked whether any of his consultant colleagues were following his example this surgeon replied that they thought he was mad. This is a sad reflection on their lack of concern about the communication needs of their patients.

6. FEEDBACK

When only verbal information has been given, the patient should be asked to repeat back to the doctor at least the essential items in the discussion. In this way understanding can be checked and repetition re-inforces learning (31). This is seldom done for it takes time but is well worthwhile. At a recent oncology clinic a patient saw a new doctor for longer than usual. When he came out the other patients in the waiting room asked him why he had been so long. 'I dunno', he said, 'the doctor kept talking to me and I kept nodding my head but I haven't a clue what he was talking about.'

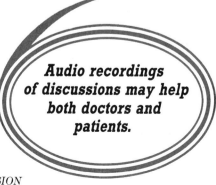

Audio recordings of discussions may help both doctors and patients.

A valuable form of feedback is for doctors to record their discussions on audio-tape so that they can listen to them afterwards and find out ways in which they could improve them. Some doctors record whole discussions and give the tapes to their patients to take home and play on their own recorders. This allows them to remind themselves, at leisure, of what the doctor had told them, in surroundings less alarming and strange to them than the clinic where they first heard them. They can then also make notes of any points which they would like doctors to explain further at their next attendance (51).

7. JARGON

This can be a major barrier to understanding between patients and doctors and should be carefully avoided in their discussions. Listening to recordings of discussions is the best way of learning how many long, obscure words one is using. Doctors are usually quite unaware of how much jargon they use in talking with patients. For example, 'making a definitive diagnosis' slips out so easily but would be better expressed as 'finding out just what is wrong with you'. Discussion of what simpler words could be used for medical terms and jargon may be profitable with groups of students. Doctors must recognise the strange ideas that patients may have about their own anatomy, their symptoms, and even the diagnoses which they report (35,36,37); but in attempting to avoid jargon adults must not be talked to as if they are children.

Continuing communication

An initial consultation is usually followed by treatment or further investigation in the course of which, especially if it is prolonged or requires admission to hospital, good communication must be maintained so that the patient remains content with what is being done and does not develop fresh anxiety or depression of which the doctor may be unaware.

Discussions at subsequent visits to a GP or to a hospital clinic and at the frequent ward visits by hospital doctors should be handled as in the initial one, except when new symptoms or other problems develop. Then good interviewing skills are needed to elucidate them. There are some special aspects to these follow-up discussions which must be attended to, particularly with in-patients.

> *Sometimes doctors talk to each other, or to a nurse, across patients' beds almost as if they were inanimate objects.*

1. GOOD MANNERS AT THE BEDSIDE

Possibly because doctors and nurses are 'in charge' of patients in hospital they sometimes tend to treat them as inferiors. Junior and senior medical staff on their rounds commonly remain standing at the beside talking down to supine and often undressed patients to their natural embarrassment (52). Sometimes doctors talk to each other or to a nurse across patients' beds, referring to them in the third person almost as if they were inanimate objects. They, and the nurses, may annoy patients by treating them almost as children (53), and nowadays they often use first names without permission. This may be all right with young patients but can upset older people. Some doctors do not even greet patients when they come to see them. Bad manners of this sort are as unacceptable in a clinical as in a social setting.

An interesting finding in one study was that when several doctors each talked to different patients at the bedside for the same time and said the same things. Half of them sat down: the others stood up. The patients thought that the sitting doctors had spent more time with them and were more interested and concerned with their welfare than those who stood up (54). However brief their visit to in-patients doctors should sit down to talk with them.

2. PREVENTING AND MANAGING PATIENTS' ANXIETIES OR DEPRESSION

Several studies of hospital in-patients have found that some 20 per cent of them already have or develop distressing anxiety or depression usually about the nature and consequences of their illnesses. Medical and nursing staff tend to under-estimate the frequency and severity of this psychological distress (11,55). Doctors, especially the junior staff who see each patient frequently, should look out for it. The results of investigations about which patients have not been told are a common cause of anxiety, for they tend to assume that no news is bad news

(56,57). They may also worry about all sorts of things they may have overheard which may have nothing to do with them. They are usually eager to know about their progress and if no one tells them about it they may fear the worst. Housemen and nurses who see patients most often should make sure that every patient is kept well informed about progress. Patients also like to know about reasons for changes in their treatment. After discharge, one patient said: 'You were treated like a child, as if it was nothing to do with you if the medicine was changed. No reason was given' (58).

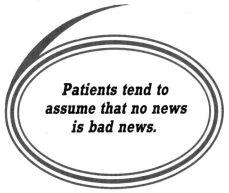

Patients tend to assume that no news is bad news.

One good technique is to encourage patients to write down their queries and worries so that they remember to ask housemen or consultants about them on their rounds (59). Many patients are alarmed by consultants' rounds. After them, a visit to each patient by nurse or houseman, can discover and allay unwarranted fears and misunderstandings. Another good tip for housemen is to visit some patients in the ward just after the lights have been turned off. People worry most when trying to get to sleep. A tactful, encouraging enquiry at this time: 'Is there anything you are worrying about?' has been found to be valuable by those who have tried it, in order to dispel unwarranted anxiety. Medical social workers can help with social worries.

A pre-operative visit by the anaesthetist has been shown not only to lessen patients' fears, but also to reduce the need for post-operative pain killers and to hasten recovery (60).

3. PATIENTS' UNAWARENESS OF
WHAT THEY HAVE BEEN TOLD

It has been reported that most patients soon forget a large proportion of what doctors tell them (31), but the methods used in these studies have now been challenged as being biased against the patient. In a recent survey of 1300 consultations by GPs it was found that when interviewed at home shortly afterwards 94 per cent of patients correctly recalled the key points of what the doctor had told them (4). So it seems that sheer forgetfulness may not be as important as had been thought in this field of medicine, where many problems are fairly simple and for much of which doctors and patients use a common terminology.

Studies of hospital patients, however, have shown that they are often ignorant of what they have been told about their diagnosis and management. Consultants have found that when

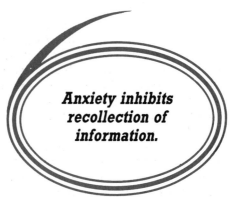

Anxiety inhibits recollection of information.

Continuing communication

they have gone to great pains to explain things simply, patients have subsequently denied having been told anything about their illnesses (61,62). The strange things that some patients say that doctors have told them (39) show how poor their understanding can be. Many patients in hospital are frightened that they may be found to have some serious disease. Anxiety inhibits recollection, particularly of complex topics. Information given on a ward round in the presence of several doctors is difficult for patients to take in. One nursing sister finds it necessary to visit all her patients after each consultant's round to relieve their frequent anxieties, and to expand upon what the consultant had meant to convey to them (63).

One way of overcoming this amnesia, induced by anxiety, would be for junior staff to discover, as should be done in the initial discussion, what the patient's hopes and fears are about the topic to be discussed and to ensure that any misunderstandings have been corrected. When this is done, immediate and later feedback of what the patient has actually taken in should be obtained so that any mistakes can be corrected and questions arising from them answered.

4. SUPERVISION OF MEDICATION

Few doctors check up carefully on their patients' compliance with treatment. Regular, friendly, and uncensorious enquiry (e.g. 'Do you find any difficulty in taking your medicines at the right times?') can detect failures and enable the doctor to give any further advice on how to comply. Giving hospital patients their own medication to take themselves at the right times, for a few days before discharge rather than continuing to have it handed out by nurses, can test understanding and thus promote correct treatment after discharge (64).

5. CONFLICTING INFORMATION

This is a problem both in hospital and family practice. Different doctors or other health professionals may be responsible. Those concerned with the patient's management have to agree on a common policy of information. One way of avoiding confusion is to have an 'information sheet' in the case notes on which questions asked by patients and answers given by staff are briefly summarised. Some trials of such sheets have failed, probably owing to insufficient preparation of staff, but they have for long been a routine part of the case notes at one hospice where they have proved an effective means of ensuring consistent communication with patients.

Lifelong illnesses

There are now many chronic illnesses which patients have to learn to control themselves under guidance from their doctors, of which insulin dependent diabetes is an example. People with this condition have to understand the nature of diabetes and how to regulate its treatment by balancing the effects of insulin and diet on blood glucose levels. They have to recognise, treat, and prevent hypoglycaemia. They also have to learn how to measure their own blood glucose to check that they are keeping it as normal as possible to avoid the grave consequences of ill-controlled diabetes. Some succeed in all this, but many fail. To doctors' surprise an inverse relationship has been found between knowledge about diabetes and its control: those with more knowledge having, on average, worse control than those who know less (65). It is now recognized that these failures of control usually have psychological causes. There may be resentment at having developed a serious disease and having to learn a lot about it, feelings of guilt and inability to cope, dislike of dependency on health professionals and disbelief in the need for scrupulous control. Rigid dieting is socially inconvenient. Some diabetologists are unaware of how cruel it can be to expect diabetics to handle all their problems with no more than strict instructions

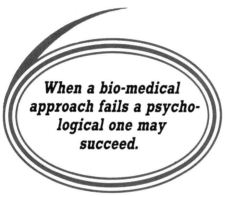

When a bio-medical approach fails a psychological one may succeed.

enforced by threats of complications. Frequent and caring support with friendly discussion is essential for these patients if they are to learn how to accept and cope with their predicaments. When this is done, control may improve markedly. A pure bio-medical approach is inadequate; a psychological one is more likely to succeed (66,67). In asthma it has also been found that just giving information about treatment increases knowledge but may not reduce morbidity (68). Here and in many other diseases requiring detailed understanding for effective control, psychological problems similar to those of the diabetic must be resolved for optimum management.

When things go wrong

Unexpected complications, particularly of hospital treatment, can cause deep distress to patients and their families. The sometimes exaggerated, wish fulfilling confidence of the public in the effectiveness of modern treatment may lead patients to have unreal expectations of success. To them failure raises suspicion of medical mistakes or incompetence. This makes it all the more important that they and their families should be given realistic and not over-optimistic information about any treatment proposed for them. Valid consent by patients is always necessary. This can only be given on the basis of effective information which must be checked by feedback to ensure that it has been understood. Patients must be told about the chances for success and about possible complications and side-effects which may arise. If treatment fails or an unexpected, serious complication occurs, this must be quickly and openly discussed with patient and family by a senior doctor who should recognize that they probably have their own intelligent, but often incorrect, views about what has happened. These must be ascertained and revised if complainers are to be satisfied with what they have been told.

Apart from the need to satisfy the patient and family, a serious consequence of failure to be frank is a doctor's appearance in court to defend an action taken by a patient. Failure to keep patients informed of what is happening to them is now one cause of an alarming rise in litigation against doctors. This usually happens because treatment has been prescribed or operations

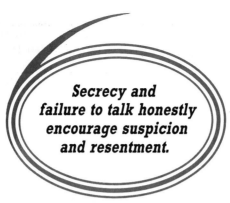

*Secrecy and
failure to talk honestly
encourage suspicion
and resentment.*

performed without explanation and without
telling patients of possible choices between
treatments or what the benefits and any risks
may be (69). If something does go wrong, all that
patients and relatives usually want is an explanation. Secrecy and failure to talk honestly
about what is happening encourages suspicion
and resentment.

Talking with the patient's family

The whole family is usually concerned when
any one of them is ill. Doctors may be so
concerned with their patient's management that
they forget to talk with other members of the
family to prevent them having misguided or
unnecessary worries and to ensure any special
help or encouragement which the patient may
need during convalescence.

The principles and skills of communication
with the family are the same as those of
communication with patients, but the sort of
things that have to be said may differ (70).

Students need to be shown how to do this by being given opportunities to talk with the families of patients they are looking after in the wards. This may be done in special sessions (71), by arranging for students, during their clinical training, to be present when the junior or senior medical staff, or the social worker talks with the families of their allocated patients. Video-tape sessions with real or simulated patients' relatives may also be used.

Listening and talking to children

With children the principles of good interviewing are similar to those with adults, for much of it has to be done with the parents, especially the mother, while including the child, particularly at the beginning of the interview and to confirm and check what the mother has said (72). Toys must be available to keep the child happy while the mother is being interviewed and the toys themselves may be used to help the child to explain symptoms (73). Children may provide information very candidly and sometimes do this better in the absence of a parent. Video-tape training has been found to be invaluable in teaching paediatric interviewing (74) and in teaching students how to handle distressed or angry parents (75). Children are often brought to the paediatrician not for the presenting problem but for what has been called 'the hidden agenda' which is a second problem related to the first which the mother will not mention without probing, but which must be dealt with if she is to be satisfied with the consultation (76).

The discussion seems to have been studied even less in paediatrics than in adult medicine. If children are told what is wrong with them with the help of illustrative drawings it is likely that parents will also better understand the nature of the illness. Indeed, medical students might well be taught how to avoid jargon by training sessions with children. As with adults, the warmth of the doctor-patient relationship, and giving a clear explanation of the diagnosis and causes of the child's illness are important in assuring compliance with treatment (77). The needs of and methods for more research into improved communication with children and their parents are the same as they are for adults.

Reassurance (78,79)

This is what many patients need to maintain their morale, but often fail to obtain. Only a doctor who is confident and interested in the patient as a person can give it: he must also be trusted and understand exactly what the patient

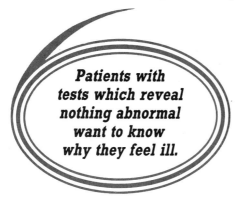

Patients with tests which reveal nothing abnormal want to know why they feel ill.

wants reassuring about. Bland dismissal of abnormality—'You're all right'—is useless, even insulting, for a patient who feels unwell. To say that a critical test is normal may be taken by the patient just to show that the wrong test has been done. Patients need to understand why they feel ill. When patients are found to have a disease which they fear, it is essential that any false ideas of its consequences should be countered. They may need help to accept their illness, so that they are willing to co-operate in its management, confident that this will restore them to well-being. On subsequent visits to such patients it may be helpful to ask 'How are you coping? Any questions?', and to make time to listen and reply. Doctors have to learn various ways of reassuring and to use what is appropriate. The essence is to concentrate on the positive aspect of recovery and retained function, not on the negative aspect of what may be lost. The patient must be told that, whatever he may have to go through, the doctor will stand by him. That, after all, is the medical contract.

Talking with patients who have fatal illnesses

This is an aspect of discussions which all students and many of their teachers find particularly difficult. Death is often a taboo subject in our society and it is the fashion to ignore its inevitable relevance to each one of us. Since doctors have to deal with many patients who are near to death, their education must include full discussion and experience of how to help these patients.

Several publications in recent years will help many teachers who are uncertain how to handle these patients with empathy (80–87). Every patient's needs are different, but a few principles may be stated about what students need to learn.

Students should be helped to escape from their own death taboo, discussing it amongst themselves with awareness of their own mortality so that they can talk to dying patients with equanimity. They should recognize that many of these patients want to know more about their outlook than doctors are ready to tell them (80,81). A simple enquiry: 'Are you worried about how you're getting on?' may give a patient a chance to speak of his fears or to show he has none (81,82).

Students need to learn the different ways in which many patients with fatal illnesses pass through states of denial, anger, resentment, depression and, with help, finally attain acceptance and peace. They must be ready to discover any unexpressed anxiety especially about terminal suffering and to relieve it by explaining that nowadays this can almost always be alleviated. They must know how successful the pharmacological and psychological management of terminal distress can be (88).

Students should be able to witness a skilled teacher enabling patients to talk by simple encouragement and to see how to handle and relieve anxiety. This may most easily be done through video-tape recordings. They should realize that 'most dying patients are far more eager for us to know what they think than that we should tell them what we think' (86).

Students must realize that there are no rules except that hope must never be extinguished (81). The alternatives are not merely silent, bland denial or stark, fatal truth. There are

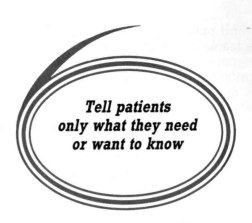

*Tell patients
only what they need
or want to know*

many degrees of truth just as there are many ways of imparting it. We have to try to learn how to give individuals what they need at any moment, in the simplest and kindest ways we can offer it, leaving them the choice to take it or leave it as they wish. Since no prognosis is precise, no patient can be told the exact truth. Rather they should be told, but only if it is clear that they want it, the most optimistic version of the future that can honestly be given. This may be difficult for students, for they often do not know what the outlook is. They must be helped here. If students are told to take histories from patients with fatal illnesses they must be forewarned that the patient may ask about prognosis and be advised how to reply.

Much suffering may be caused by casual misstatements or hints of an inevitable fatal outcome. It is always essential to maintain the patient's morale.

Students must also be made aware of the importance of communicating with the family, telling them no more than is absolutely necessary. Distress can be caused if patients sense that their families know something that is being kept from them.

Finally students need guidance about how to

assuage the distress of the bereaved. Role playing sessions under guidance can be helpful both here and in other aspects of talking with patients who have serious disease.

Research into how to communicate better with patients

Studies of doctor's communication skills have hitherto concentrated almost entirely on the interview and we now know the common errors that students make and how they may learn to avoid them so that they continue to interview well after qualification (5). Recent studies of communication in general practice have extended this to indicate how doctors can discuss their advice with patients better (4,15). We now need to discover how widely these methods are being used in primary care and how any desirable improvements could be brought about.

At present we know practically nothing about the communication skills of consultants who do most of the teaching of students. Here there are many opportunities for teachers to encourage each other, or their juniors, to do controlled trials of various methods, verbal, written, or recorded, to see how these could be used to promote patient satisfaction and therapeutic effectiveness. The methods which have shown how consultations in general practice can be improved (4,15) should be tested in hospital practice where they should be equally beneficial. The value of the model presented in Appendix 2 needs testing in both areas of practice. Such studies are best done in collaboration with social psychologists who can better appreciate the patient's point of view and needs better than can doctors. It is to be hoped that these kinds of research, which can be relatively inexpensive, will be more vigorously prosecuted in the future than they are at present.

Timing and testing of communication teaching (89)

In many medical schools behavioural and psychological aspects of encounters between people are discussed with advantage in the pre-clinical period, but clinical interviewing skills are best taught by video feedback when students first have to talk with patients on their own, often at the beginning of the first clinical year. It has been found that if they are taught before they meet patients regularly, these skills may not persist (90). Most medical students already have social skills which are appropriate to clinical interviewing. Helping students to identify those skills which they do or do not possess can form a good basis for clinical teaching.

Teaching the discussion is better left until students have enough medical knowledge to feel confident in telling patients and their families about diagnosis and management. Every medical school should ensure that this teaching is done by video feedback so that students can see for themselves what they are doing wrong and be helped to become more competent. The importance of doctors listening and talking to patients in ways which will help them to talk freely, and of using simple language which they

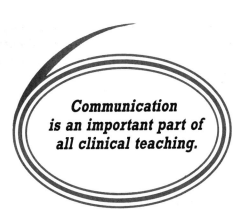

Communication is an important part of all clinical teaching.

can understand, needs to be stressed throughout clinical teaching. Allocation of curriculum time for this teaching will enable formal teaching and permit its evaluation, thus emphasising its importance to students. All clinical teachers should make opportunities to monitor and foster these essential skills and should not leave such teaching only to those who express a special interest. It should be noted that the General Medical Council is now becoming more concerned about these needs (91).

At present these skills, so essential to the effective practice of medicine, are not tested at the time of the final professional examination, although at least one medical school is planning to include them (92). There are considerable logistic difficulties in arranging for the video assessment which would be necessary, but it should be possible to overcome them, and all medical schools should be planning how best to do this. Assessment of video-tapes could be done by trained psychologists who might better appreciate the patient's point of view, which is of primary importance in doctor-patient communication.

The problem would remain of what should be done about those candidates who, though having sufficient clinical knowledge, lack any ability to communicate effectively with patients. Some might be enabled to improve with psychological help, others might need advice to enter some non-clinical branch of medicine.

Special Considerations

(93)

Patients with special problems

---

1. FOREIGNERS

Communication with patients from another culture is often difficult (94). If they share no language with the doctor a fluent interpreter is essential for verbal communication, but the usual non-verbal expressions of interest and concern should be used. Speak slowly, clearly and quietly, looking at the patient, not the interpreter. Explain your aims in both interview and discussion to the interpreter who may have to amplify what you say. It is particularly difficult to deal with psycho-social problems and easy to assume that those who speak English well think as we do and to overlook any confusion that may be occurring.

Death and bereavement are thought of and managed differently in certain foreign ethnic groups in Britain and their wishes and fears should be carefully attended to (95).

2. DEAF PATIENTS

The first thing is to be sure that the patient has a hearing aid. In some hospitals high fidelity aids are available. Without aids, deaf patients may be helped by putting a stethoscope into their ears and speaking directly into the chest piece. If you have to speak very loud try not to sound angry. Most deaf people learn—in varying degrees—to lip read. Try speaking quietly but slowly, enunciating every word clearly; good lighting and an unobstructed full face view at a distance of 3–4 feet are essential for normal lip movements to be seen clearly. Look directly at the patient. If the patient does not understand a question, rephrase it more simply, if that fails, write it down. In any case write down instructions for treatment (96).

3. PATIENTS WITH SPEECH PROBLEMS

These may be of many kinds, chiefly various forms of neurological disorder, but also of mental deficiency. People who cannot talk freely may understand speech normally and are most annoyed if they are addressed in baby language. The handicapped are quick to note non-verbal indicators of lack of concern or respect. They should be addressed in terms appropriate to their age, using simple words and not speaking too fast. Longer pauses than usual should be left for answers to questions, which may be rephrased and asked again if they are not understood (97).

Health education

The communication skills hitherto discussed relate mainly to the diagnostic and therapeutic aspects of a consultation. But this is also an occasion for helping patients not only to get well, but also to keep well, by telling them how they may avoid recurrences of their present illness. This can be extended to give general advice about what they could do to be less likely to develop illnesses of other kinds. The trouble about this sort of advice is that it usually involves telling people not to do things that they want to do (smoking, drinking—especially before driving—eating rich foods) or to do things they don't want to do (taking more exercise, submitting to various screening procedures and even behaving better in their families).

There is some debate about the responsibility of doctors in this area (98,99). On the one hand it can be effective because of the unique, trustful

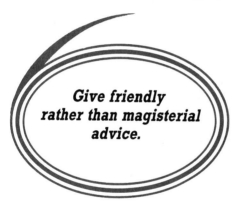

Give friendly rather than magisterial advice.

relationship between doctor and patient; on the other hand it alters the doctor's traditional role from a provider of services to those who ask for them to one in which unrequested advice is given. On the whole the latter role is accepted because it is generally beneficial and many patients now expect it from their doctors. In both primary and hospital care doctors should seek out and use suitable occasions to persuade patients to adopt healthy and to eschew harmful habits. This can be more effectively done by doctors who have followed their own advice.

The methods to be used in this aspect of a doctor's work are the same as those already suggested for the conduct of a discussion, but it is particularly important to enquire about habits in an unreproachful manner so as to encourage telling the truth and to give friendly rather than magisterial advice. When this has been done a note should be made in the patient's record and follow-up questions asked on subsequent visits to reinforce the message.

APPENDIX 1

A model for a clinical interview

The model for an interview which follows is abbreviated from that described by Maguire and Rutter (16). This is an outstanding paper which many teachers may wish to read in full. Others may find the seven task model of Pendleton *et al* (15) more helpful, or the 20 objectives listed by Crisp (89).

The main purpose of providing a model is to avoid students creating an inappropriate one for themselves during their clinical work. They tend to adopt either an 'organic' stance or a 'psychiatric' one, neither of which alone will match their patients' needs.

A model needs consistent logic to be remembered by the interviewer and appreciated by patients. This permits an approach to intimate questions which may be asked without seeming to make an unnecessary invasion of personal privacy. It also shows the range of data which students should have collected at the end of the interview.

THE MODEL

1. *Nature of the current problems*

The doctor must first help the patient with an entirely open question such as 'What's your problem?' and listen attentively to whatever problem the patient volunteers. Some patients first mention a physical symptom when their main problems are social or psychological; so the doctor should always ask if there are any other problems the patient would like to mention, for there may be several. If the doctor then summarises his understanding of the problem(s), the patient can be offered a further opportunity to expand upon or add to them. If there seem to be too many to deal with in the time available the doctor should agree with the patient which one should be dealt with on this first occasion, offering a further occasion to deal with the others.

2. *Details of the (selected) current problems*

For each problem the following information is needed:—

(i) Date and time of onset, usually by relating it to some social event.

(ii) Subsequent development, noting change points and associated events or activities.

(iii) Precipitating or relieving factors which may be as general as 'overwork' or as specific as 'eating pickled onions'. People tend to account for problems by blaming recent events. The doctors should not accept these apparent correlations without careful dating.

(iv) Full details and times of treatment already taken.

3. *Impact of the problems on patient and family*

(i) Serious effects on the day-to-day functioning of the patient and his family are often not volunteered and should be asked about; also:

(ii) Availability of support, particularly from close relatives in both practical and emotional terms.

4. *Patients' views of their problems*

Two aspects need to be considered here.

First, patients' pre-conceptions about diagnosis and treatment should be elucidated. If these conflict with the doctor's ideas, clear reasons should be given for accepting the doctor's in preference to the patient's. At present few patients think that their ideas will interest doctors so they are reluctant to mention them for fear of being thought stupid. Others may want to leave it all to the doctor and won't say anything unless they are sure the doctor is wrong. Getting round these difficulties demands an easy doctor-patient relationship.

Second, any anxieties that patients may have must be discovered. Specific questions about fears of cancer or heart disease and, if depressed, about thoughts of suicide should be asked.

(For a full discussion of this part of the interview see reference 4, 269–72).

5. *Pre-disposition to illness*

Questions should be asked about smoking, alcohol abuse, diet, and drug taking, and also about previous physical or psychological illnesses. These will lead on to:

6. *Screening questions*

These are used to check that no relevant symptoms have been overlooked. When an interview has focussed mainly on organic problems the screening questions might focus on changes of mood and *vice versa*. This enquiry can often be made during the physical examination.

APPENDIX 2
A model for the discussion

Discussion with patients range from a few words of re-assurance to longer conversations on several occasions. The model which follows is intended to cover many situations (but not a course of counselling) so it has to be more elaborate than that of the interview. It is at least a reminder of strategies which, although often omitted, are necessary if discussions are to satisfy patients and lead to effective management.

A satisfactory discussion requires that you should have made at least a provisional diagnosis of the patient's main problem. To simplify the model it will be assumed that you have diagnosed a single problem. Other problems can be discussed in the same way later.

Before telling patients your diagnosis and proposals for treatment you should ask them (if you have not already done this in the interview) what they believe or fear may be wrong with them and what treatment they expect. This should reveal any unwarranted anxieties or misconceptions which can be dealt with immediately. If they have no such ideas or they agree with yours the discussion can proceed on this basis. If they prefer their own ideas you should explain clearly and simply why you disagree. This will usually lead to some conclusion which will satisfy the patient. Sometimes an investigation, such as an X-ray, will be needed to alleviate a patient's fears.

INVESTIGATIONS

When these are needed begin by saying 'We shall need to do some tests to check what is wrong

with you. Would you like to know about them?'
If the answer is 'Yes', as is usually the case, take
each investigation (which the patient has not
previously had) and explain for each:

1. Its purpose.
2. What will actually be done to the patient.
3. Any discomfort it may cause.
4. How soon the result will be known.
5. How the patient will be told about this.

Then ask how the patient feels about the tests.
Any fears should be explored and truthful
reassurance given. Ask if there are any further
questions and answer them honestly without
minimizing common difficulties.

DIAGNOSIS, PROGNOSIS AND CAUSES

1. *Uncertain diagnosis*

Sometimes, particularly in primary care, it is
impossible to make a definite diagnosis. It is
then best to be honest with the patient by
saying, for example, 'I don't know what is wrong
with you, but I'm sure it's not serious. Please
come and see me again if you don't soon feel
better'. This kind of condition has been described as 'temporary dependency' (100) and has
a good prognosis with firm re-assurance (101).

2. *Physical illness with good prognosis*

This can often be diagnosed confidently on
clinical grounds, but may need confirmation by
investigations. When the diagnosis has been
made the patient should be told:

a. **A name.** Patients like to have a name for
their illness to tell family or friends what is
wrong with them. Ask what the patient thinks
the name means and if this is wrong, correct it.
Simple medical words have quite different
meanings for laymen and doctors (35–37). If the

diagnosis is still unproven but may be grave, don't name what you fear but give an indication such as 'inflammation of the nerves' rather than 'multiple sclerosis'.

b. **Its cause.** If this is unknown, means for avoiding recurrence should be discussed. If it is unknown, as it often is, admit this but accept patients' harmless ideas ('Yes, could be').

c. **The prognosis.** If the good prognosis depends upon effective treatment make sure that the patient has understood this and will carry out the treatment; for cure or control depends on it. This can be checked by a question such as, 'I hope you accept that you will be O.K. Is there anything more you want to know about the treatment?' See below for handling of more complex long-term controllable illnesses.

3. *Physical illness with poor prognosis*

This is usually known only after hospital investigation. The specialist, who may have given a hint of serious illness should ask, 'When we have all the results would you like me to tell you about them or would you prefer to discuss them with your GP, to whom I shall send them?' This question has been found to distinguish those, usually about 50 per cent, who want to know if they have a fatal cancer from those who do not (103).

If it falls to you to give bad news to a patient the truth should be approached gradually. At first say something like, 'I'm afraid it's not a simple ulcer, it looks more serious'. You can temporise again with, 'The biopsy showed a few abnormal cells'. The patient who wants more information may ask, 'Do you mean it's cancer?' In answer to this direct question patients should be asked what the word means to them and be told how many types can be cured or controlled.

The issue must not be shirked as many doctors do (104). It must be handled with honesty and optimism to prevent persistence of unjustified fears of rapid death and unrelieved suffering.

Patients and their families are always grateful for a more favourable prognosis than what is indicated clinically. One widow whose elderly husband in heart failure had been told, truthfully, that he might not live more than two years, said to the physician after his death, 'How could you do what you did to my husband? For him the past two years have been a living death'. The truth may, of course, be needed by patients with financial commitments, but should be given to them with sensitivity.

The principles of discussing fatal illnesses are further described on p. 40.

4. *Psychiatric illness*

Tell the patient:

a. **A name.** Indicate that this is a well recognized illness which has no more serious implications than any physical illness. Then explore how the patient has responded to the diagnosis and deal with any particular worries about the outcome and long-term prognosis.

b. **Its cause(s).** It is helpful to explore the patient's ideas of causes by asking, 'Why do you think you have become ill just now?' You can then discuss your own views of the causes and move towards an agreement about what the most important factors have been. This may require further discussions on other occasions because psychiatric patients are especially eager to find a meaning for their illnesses and may seize on irrelevant recent events.

THERAPY

A. **Treatments to be carried out by patients themselves**

Before discussing treatment the doctor should make sure that the patient wants it. Sometimes they want to manage their problems themselves or to seek 'alternative' therapy. If the doctor considers rejection of the proposed treatment unwise it is important to ensure that the patient understands the probable consequences.

1. *Simple drug therapy*

Ask women of child-bearing age if they might be pregnant. If so, some drugs must be avoided. Ideally, each patient should be told for each medicine:

 1. Its name.

 2. What it is intended to do—control or cure?

 3. Dose and frequency.

 4. To be taken before or after meals—how long?

 5. How to take it. If orally, to be swallowed with at least 3 oz of water.

 6. How long to go on taking it. Importance of completing the course even if symptoms disappear.

 7. Any special precautions (e.g. before driving or using machinery).

 8. Any interactions with other drugs, foods, or alcohol.

 9. Possible side effects and what to do if they occur. Patient to ask doctor or pharmacist if uncertain whether symptoms are due to the medicine.

 10. Storage (out of reach of children). In fridge?

11. Disposal of any excess (tablets down toilet). Canisters not to be thrown into fire.

12. What to do if a dose is missed or extra one(s) taken.

13. How to tell if the medicine is working and what to do if it isn't.

14. Any subsequent questions to be asked of doctor or pharmacist.

This is a lot of information to be given in a consultation or for patients to remember without writing it down. At present this is the best thing for them to do. Pharmaceutical companies are preparing to supply patient information leaflets with all prescriptions and a compendium of them will be published. You will then be able to discuss these leaflets with patients. This will be particularly important with patients who are illiterate, blind or cannot read English. They will have to be given the information verbally by you or by a friend who can tell them what the leaflets say.

2. *More complex therapy*

With or without special diets or use of equipment which require active management by patients themselves with monitoring of effects e.g. asthma, diabetes, renal dialysis. These patients need instruction extending over weeks or months from nurses, dieticians, and other health professionals. Doctors must understand and sympathise with patients' shock and distress when they are told the diagnosis. Firm reassurance should be given that they will really be able to cope. Effective support by specialist nurses as well as by doctors must be maintained as these patients set about learning the necessary skills which, when acquired and used diligently, will enable them to live essentially normal lives. They should be told about patients' associations through which they can meet and discuss their problems with others who have the same disability (48,49).

3. *Changes in daily activities (lifestyle)*

1. Job: Continue as before.
   Stay off work temporarily (state period).
   Change job. Reach agreement through reflective questions*.

2. Exercise: Avoid, reduce, continue or increase.
   Be precise e.g. 'Brisk walk for at least 30 minutes daily'.
   Bedrest: state how long, how complete.

3. Diet: Foods to be increased or decreased.
   Refer to dietician if strict diet needed.

4. Sex: If impaired by illness, suggest what to do or whom to consult.

5. Tobacco: If smoker, firm advice to stop. If too difficult, try nicotine gum.

6. Alcohol: Enquire about consumption without disapproval.
   If excessive, point out dangers to self and others.
   If reduction needed, give specific daily limit.
   If to be stopped, consider reference to helping agency (49, pp. 13–15).

B. **Therapy to be carried out by health professionals** (e.g. operations, radio-therapy, physio-therapy).

First say what is proposed (e.g. remove gall stone, put in new hip, X-ray or chemotherapy of lump). Then ask patients how much they want to know. Some will, in effect, say 'I don't want

---

* e.g. if patient asks: 'Should I change my job?', reply 'What do *you* think about that?'

A model for the discussion

any details; I leave it to you to get me well'. Others may want to know more before agreeing to treatment. At an initial consultation full details will not usually be needed but the following information should be given, including:

1. Control or cure? Use statements such as: 'I'm sure it will get rid of your problem'; 'We should get it under control'; 'It should slow the process down'.

2. Any unpleasant side effects. For surgery, how much it will hurt.

3. Any consequent long-term disability. Ask if patients agree to have the treatment. They may want to go away and think about it. After agreement tell them:

4. Where treatment will be done—in-patient or out-patient.

5. When it will be done. If long waiting list, discuss going to District with shorter waiting list (102).

6. How long it will take. If the patient rejects the proposed treatment or there will be long delay, advise (as in A.1 above) alternative or interim treatment while waiting for the principal therapy.

INFORMED CONSENT TO TREATMENT (105)

Treatment must be explained clearly, without jargon, so that as far as possible informed consent can be given. Consent to simple drug therapy is usually implied by the patient agreeing to it during the discussion and a note of this should be put into the case record. When the treatment has risks, signed consent similar to that obtained from patients before surgery should be obtained. Do not suppose that a signature implies comprehension (106) so always make sure that patients understand what is to be done and that it is their choice to start or to stop the treatment if they find any of its effects intolerable: the responsibility is theirs.

To be sure that there has been no misunderstanding you can ask patients to repeat back to you what you have told them about the treatment. One good way of doing this is to ask in a friendly manner, 'When you get home what will you tell them I have told you about the treatment?' Any mistakes can then be rectified and the correct version preferably written down.

SOCIAL PROBLEMS

If the interview has disclosed social difficulties or unhappy personal relationships which are causing or being caused by the patient's illness they must be tackled in the discussion. In their vocational training GPs learn the means by which they can themselves solve simpler problems and the local agencies to which more difficult ones can be referred. Hospital specialists usually refer these matters to medical social workers. No matter how such problems are handled the important thing is that they should be considered in the discussion.

References

1. SPENCE, J. 'The need for understanding the individual as part of the training and function of doctors and nurses'. Reprinted in *The Purpose and Practice of Medicine*. London: Oxford University Press, 1960, pp.271–80.

2. KERR, D. N. S. 'Teaching communication skills in postgraduate medical education'. *Proc. Roy Soc. Med.*, 1986, **79**:575–80.

3. BYRNE, P. S. *Doctors talking to patients: a study of verbal behaviour of general practitioners consulting in their surgeries*. London: HMSO, 1976.

4. TUCKETT, D., *et al. Meetings between experts: an approach to sharing ideas in medical consultations*. London: Tavistock Publications, 1985.

5. MAGUIRE, P., FAIRBAIRN, S. AND FLETCHER, C. 'Consultation skills of young doctors: I. Benefits of feedback training in interviewing as students persist: II. Most young doctors are bad at giving information'. *Br. Med. J.*, 1986, **292**:1537–78.

6. HELFER, R. E. 'An objective comparison of the interviewing skills of freshmen and senior medical students'. *Paediatrics*, 1970, **45**:623–7.

7. MAGUIRE, R. P. AND RUTTER, D. R. 'History taking by medical students: 1. Deficiencies in performance. 2. Evaluation of a training programme'. *Lancet*, 1976, **2**:556–60.

8. DUFFY, D. L., HAMERMAN, D. AND COHEN, M. A. 'Communication skills of house officers: a study in a medical clinic. *Ann. Intern. Med.*, 1980, **93**:3547.

9. FELDMAN, E., *et al*. 'Psychiatric disorders in medical inpatients'. *Q. J. Med.*, 1987, **63**:405–12.

10. GOLDBERG, D. P. AND BLACKWELL, B. 'Psychiatric illness in general practice: a detailed study using a new method of case identification'. *Br. Med. J.*, 1970, **2**:439–41.

11. MAGUIRE, G. P., *et al*. 'Psychiatric morbidity and referral on two general medical wards'. *Br. Med. J.*, 1974, **1**:268–70.

12. NABARRO, J. 'Unrecognised psychiatric illness in medical patients'. *Br. Med. J.*, 1984, **289**:635–6.

13. PLATT, F. W. AND MCMATH, J. C. 'Clinical Hypocompetence: the interview'. *Ann. Intern. Med.*, 1979, **91**:898–902.

14. HAMPTON, J. R., *et al*. 'Relative contributions of history taking, physical examination and laboratory investigations to diagnosis and management of medical out-patients'. *Br. Med. J.*, 1975, **2**:486–9.

15. PENDLETON, D., *et al. The Consultation: an approach to learning and teaching.* Oxford: Oxford University Press, 1984.

16. MAGUIRE, G. P. AND RUTTER, D. R. 'Training medical students to communicate'. In BENNETT, A. E. (ed). *Communication between Doctors and Patients.* London: Oxford University Press for the Nuffield Provincial Hospitals Trust, 1979, pp.47–74.

17. MAGUIRE, G. P., *et al.* 'The value of feedback in teaching interviewing skills to medical students'. *Psych. Med.*, 1978, **8**:697–704.

18. VERBY, J. E., HOLDEN, P. AND DAVIS, R. H. 'Peer review of consultations in primary care: the use of audio-visual recordings'. *Br. Med. J.*, 1979, **1**:1686–8.

19. WAKEFORD, R. 'Communication skills training in United Kingdom medical schools'. In PENDELTON, D. AND HASLER, J. (eds). *Doctor-Patient Communication.* London: Academic Press, 1983, pp. 233–48.

20. THOMPSON, J. A. AND ANDERSON, J. L. 'Patient preferences and the bedside manner'. *Med. Educ.*, 1982, **16**:17–21.

21. BAIN, D. J. G. 'Doctor-patient communication in general practice consultations'. *Med. Educ.*, 1976, **10**:125–31.

22. JAMES, B. AND LORD, D. J. 'Human sexuality and medical education'. *Lancet*, 1976, **ii**:560–8.

23. STANLEY, E. 'An introduction to sexuality in the medical curriculum'. *Med. Educ.*, 1978, **12**:441–5.

24. ROLAND, M. O., *et al.* 'The "five minute" consultation: effect of time constraint on verbal communication'. *Br. Med. J.*, 1986, **292**:874–6.

25. HALL, G. H. 'Experience with out-patient medical questionnaires'. *Br. Med. J.*, 1972, **1**:42–5.

26. BRODY, D. S. 'The patient's role in clinical decision-making'. *Ann. Intern. Med.*, 1980, **93**:718–22.

27. SCOTT, R. B. 'The bedside manner'. *Trans. Med. Soc. Lond.*, 1965, **82**:1–12.

28. CARTWRIGHT, A. AND ANDERSON, R. *General Practice Revisited, a second study of patients and their doctors.* London: Tavistock, 1981.

29. DAVIS, A., HOROBIN, G. (eds). *Medical Encounters: the experience of illness and treatment.* London: Groom Helm, 1977.

30. DUNKELMAN, H. 'Patients' knowledge of their conditions and treatment and how it might be improved'. *Br. Med. J.*, 1979, **2**:311–4.

31. LEY, P. 'Patients' understanding and recall in clinical communication failure'. In PENDLETON, D. AND HASLER, J.

(eds). *Doctor-Patient Communication*. London: Academic Press, 1983, pp. 89–107.

32. HAYNES, R. B., TAYLOR, D. W. AND SACKETT, D. L. *Compliance in Health Care*. Baltimore and London: Johns Hopkins University Press, 1979.

33. DRURY, V. W. M., WADE, O. L. AND WOOLF, E. 'Following advice in general practice'. *J. Roy. Coll. Gen. Pract.*, 1976, **26:**712–8.

34. WAITZKIN, H. AND STOECKLE, J. D. 'The communication of information about illness'. *Adv. Psych. Med.*, 1972, **8:**180–215.

35. BOYLE, C. M. 'Difference between patients' and doctors' interpretation of some common medical terms'. *Br. Med. J.*, 1970, **2:**286–9.

36. PEARSON, J. AND DUDLEY, M. A. F. 'Bodily perceptions in surgical patients'. *Br. Med. J.*, 1982, **284:**1545–6.

37. KINGHAM, J. G. C., FAIRCLOUGH, P. D. AND DAWSON, A. M. 'What is indigestion?' *J. Roy. Soc. Med.*, 1983, **76:**183–6.

38. BARNLAND, D. C. 'The mystification of meaning: doctor-patient encounters'. *J. Med. Educ.*, 1976, **51:**716–25.

39. ASHER, R. *Talking Sense*. London: Pitman Medical, 1971, p.116.

40. FURNESS, M. E. 'Reporting obstetric ultrasound'. *Lancet*, 1987, **i:**675–6.

41. HOFFENBERG, R. *Clinical Freedom*. London: Nuffield Provincial Hospitals Trust, 1987, pp.93–4.

42. JASPARS, J., KING, J. AND PENDLETON, D. 'The consultation: a social psychological analysis'. In PENDLETON, D. AND HASLER, J. *Doctor-Patient Communication*. London: Academic Press, 1983, pp.149–51.

43. STIMPSON, G. V. 'Obeying doctors' orders: a view from the other side'. *Soc. Sci. Med.*, 1974, **8:**97–104.

44. RIDOUT, S., WATERS, W. E. AND GEORGE, C. F. 'Knowledge of and attitudes to medicines in the Southampton community'. *Br. J. Clin. Pharmac.*, 1986, **21:**701–12.

45. MORRIS, L. A. AND HALPERIN, J. A. 'Effects of written drug information on patient knowledge and compliance: a literature review'. *Am. J. Publ. Hlth.*, 1979, **69:**47–52.

46. GIBBS, S., WATERS, W. E. AND GEORGE, C. F. 'The design of prescription information leaflets and feasibility of their use in general practice'. *Pharmceut. Med.*, 1987, **2:**23–33.

47. GEORGE, C. F. 'Telling patients about their medicines'. *Br. Med. J.*, 1987, **294:**1566–7.

48. GUNN, A. D. G. 'Self-help'. *Br. Med. J.*, 1984, **288:**1024.

49. PATIENTS' ASSOCIATION. *Self-help and the patient. A directory of national organisations concerned with various diseases and handicaps*. Tenth Ed. London: Patients' Association (Room 30, 18 Charing Cross Road, WC2H 0HR) 1986.

REFERENCES

50. WELFORD, W. 'Closing the communication gap'. *Nursing Times*, 1975, January 16th.

51. BUTT, H. R. 'A method for better physician-patient communication'. *Ann. Intern. Med.*, 1977, **86**:478–80.

52. YOUNG, B. 'Anaphylaxis'. In MANDEL, M. AND SPIRO, M. *When Doctors Get Sick*. New York: Plenum Publishing Corp., 1987, pp.390–1.

53. FIRTH, R. 'Routines in a tropical diseases hospital'. In DAVIS, A. AND HOROBIN, G. (eds). *Medical Encounters: the experience of illness and treatment*. London: Groom Helm, 1977, pp.143–158.

54. ANONYMOUS. In MANDEL, M. AND SPIRO, M. (eds). *When Doctors Get Sick*. New York: Plenum Publishing Corp., 1987, p.434.

55. JOHNSTON, M. 'Communication of patients' feelings in hospital'. In BENNETT, A. E. (ed). *Communication Between Doctors and Patients*. London: Oxford University Press for Nuffield Provincial Hospitals Trust, 1976, pp.31–43.

56. HAWKINS, C. 'Patients' reactions to their investigations: a study of 504 patients'. *Br. Med. J.*, 1979, **2**:638–40.

57. REYNOLDS, M. 'No news is bad news: patients' views about communication in hospital'. *Br. Med. J.*, 1978, **1**:1673–6.

58. CARTWRIGHT, A. *Human Relations and Hospital Care*. London: Routledge and Kegan Paul, 1964, pp.73–107.

59. HAWKINS, C. *Mishap or Malpractice?* Oxford: Blackwell Scientific Publications, 1985, p.283.

60. MATTHEWS, A. AND RIDGEWAY, V. 'Psychological preparation for surgery'. In STEPTOE, A. AND MATTHEWS, A. (eds). *Health Care and Human Behavior*. London: Academic Press, 1984, pp.231–59.

61. ELLIS, D. A., HOPKIN, J. M., LEITCH, A. G. AND CROFTON, J. 'Doctors' orders: controlled trial of supplementary written information for patients'. *Br. Med. J.*, 1979, **1**:456.

62. CAMERON, I. Personal communication.

63. TIERNEY, A. Personal communication.

64. WILSON, G. M. 'Prescribing for patients leaving hospital'. *Prescr. J.*, 1972, **12**:63–8.

65. WILLIAMS, T. F., *et al.* 'The clinical picture of diabetic control studied in four settings'. *Am. J. Publ. Hlth.*, 1967, **57**:441–51.

66. ASSAL, J. P. 'A global, integrated approach to diabetis: a challenge for more efficient therapy'. In DAVIDSON, J. K. (ed). *Clinical Diabetes Mellitus. A problem-orientated approach*. New York: Thieme Inc., 1986, pp.560–73.

67. DUNN, S. M. 'Reactions to educational techniques: coping strategies for diabetes and learning'. *Diabet. Med.*, 1986, **3**:419–29.

68. Hilton, S., *et al.* 'Controlled evaluation of the effect of patient education on asthma morbidity in general practice'. *Lancet*, 1986, **i**:26–9.

69. Hawkins, C. and Paterson, I. 'Medico-legal audit in the West Midlands region: analysis of 100 cases'. *Br. Med. J.*, 1987, **295:**1533–6.

70. Brummel-Smith, K. 'Interviewing the family'. In Enelow, A. J. and Swisher, S. N. (eds) *Interviewing and Patient Care.* 3rd Ed. New York: Oxford University Press, 1986, pp.163–181.

71. Brooke, B. N. 'The clinical approach'. *Lancet*, 1960, **ii:**810–12.

72. Kahn, J. H. 'Communication with children and patients'. *Br. Med. J.*, 1972, **3:**404–8.

73. Enzer, N. B. 'Interviewing children and parents'. In Enelow, A. J. and Swisher, S. N. (eds). *Interviewing and Patient Care.* New York: Oxford University Press, 3rd ed., 1986, pp.122–47.

74. Korsch, B. M. and Negrette, V. F. 'Doctor-patient communication'. *Scien. Amer.*, 1972, **227(2):**66–71.

75. Meadow, R. and Hewitt, C. 'Teaching communication skills with the help of actresses and video-tape simulation'. *Br. J. Med. Educ.*, 1972, **6:**317–22.

76. Menahem, S. 'Teaching students of medicine to listen: the missed diagnosis from a hidden agenda'. *J. Roy. Soc. Med.*, 1987, **80:**343–6.

77. Francis, V., Korsch, B. M. and Morris, M. J. 'Gaps in the doctor-patient relationship: patients' response to medical advice'. *N. Eng. J. Med.*, 1969, **280:**535–40.

78. Kessel, N. 'Reassurance'. *Lancet*, 1979, **i:**1128–33.

79. Warwick, H. M. C. and Salkovskis, P. M. 'Reassurance'. *Br. Med. J.*, 1985, **290:**1028.

80. Bloch, S. 'Instruction on death and dying for the medical student'. *Med. Educ.*, 1976, **10:**269–73.

81. Brewin, T. B. 'The cancer patient: communication and morale'. *Br. Med. J.*, 1977, **2:**1623–27.

82. Crammond, W. A. 'Psychotherapy of the dying patient'. *Br. Med. J.*, 1970, **3:**389–93.

83. Hinton, J. *Dying.* Harmondsworth: Penguin Books, 2nd Ed., 1972.

84. Irwin, W. G. 'Teaching terminal care at Queens University of Belfast'. *Br. Med. J.*, 1984, **28:**1509–11.

85. Maclean, U. 'Learning about death'. *J. Med. Eth.*, 1979, **5:**68–70.

86. Saunders, C. M. (ed). *The Management of Terminal Disease.* London: Edward Arnold, 1978.

87. Buckman, R. *I Don't Know What to Say.* London: Papermac, 1988.

88. WALSH, T. D. AND WEST, T. S. 'Controlling symptoms in advanced cancer'. *Br. Med. J.*, 1988, **296:**477–8.

89. CRISP, A. M. 'Undergraduate training for communication in medical practice'. *J. Roy. Soc. Med.*, 1986, **79:**568–74.

90. ENGLER, C. M., SALTZMAN, G. A., WALKER, M. L. AND WOLF, E. M. 'Medical student acquisition and retention of communication and interviewing skills'. *J. Med. Educ.*, 1981, **56:**572–9.

91. McCORMICK, J. 'Communication skills'. *J. Roy. Soc. Med.*, 1986, **79:**563.

92. BARBER, J. H. University of Glasgow, Department of General Practice. Personal Communication.

93. FLETCHER, C. 'Listening and talking to patients: some special problems. *Br. Med. J.*, 1980, **281:**1056–8.

94. BAL, P. 'Communication with non-English-speaking patients'. *Br. Med. J.*, 1981, **283:**368–9.

95. BLACK, J. 'How to do it: broaden your mind about death and bereavement in certain ethnic groups in Britain'. *Br. Med. J.*, 1987, **295:**536–8.

96. DICKINSON, T. 'Communicating with deaf patients'. *Br. Med. J.*, 1981, **282:**544–5.

97. THRUSH, J. 'Communicating with patients with speech or language problems'. *Br. Med. J.*, 1981, **282:**802–3,878–9.

98. GILLON, R. 'Health education and health promotion'. *J. Med. Eth.*, 1987, **13:**3–4.

99. TOON, P. D. 'Promoting prevention and patient autonomy: discussion paper'. *J. Roy. Soc. Med.*, 1987, **80:**502–4.

100. THOMAS, K. B. 'Temporarily dependent patient in general practice'. *Br. Med. J.*, 1974, **1:**625–6.

101. THOMAS, K. B. 'General practice consultations: is there any point in being positive?' *Br. Med. J.*, 1987, **294:**1200–2.

102. COLLEGE OF HEALTH. *Hospital Waiting Lists.* London: College of Health, 18 Victoria Park Square, London E2 9PF.

103. SPENCER-JONES, J. 'Telling the right patient'. *Br. Med. J.*, 1981, **283:**291–2.

104. MAGUIRE, P. 'Barriers to the psychological care of the dying'. *Br. Med. J.*, 1985, **291:**1711–3.

105. KING, J. 'Informed consent. A review of the empirical evidence'. *IME Bulletin,* Suppl. 3, Dec 1986.

106. BYRNE, D. J., NAPIER, A. AND CUSCHIERI, A. 'How informed is signed consent?' *Br. Med. J.*, 1988, **296:**839–40.

NOTES

NOTES

NOTES

NOTES